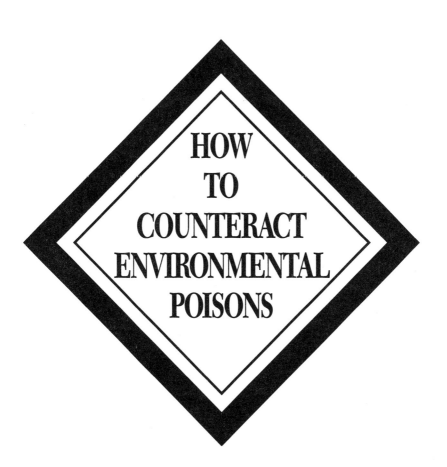

HOW
TO
COUNTERACT
ENVIRONMENTAL
POISONS

A Collection of Teachings
by Hanna Kroeger

How to Counteract Environmental Poisons

3rd Printing, 1996

ISBN 1-883713-15-3

Introduction

This book is a collection of ideas given to us by Reverend Hanna Kroeger, Minister of the Chapel of Miracles in Boulder, Colorado. She has written many books helping us with our physical and spiritual needs. Now it is time for us to protect our homes and our families. Jesus said: "Keep my house clean until I return." There are simple, quick procedures to protect us from all negative energy, dark forces and poisons that can ruin our health and destroy our families. Your health and well-being are in your own hands. The pressure of despair brings about inventions and new help, but you must seek it out and apply it. Not your government, not your physician, but you, and you alone, will be able to protect your beloved ones and yourself.

Many of these procedures require you to do something. This accomplishes two things. First, your faith, your obedience, your willingness to help yourself, to take the initiative, opens the door to Christ. Secondly, the task, the procedure, the object you've made, will do its part to protect and heal you also. When you do something in the physical, good or bad, it affects the spiritual, and when you do something spiritual, it affects the physical. The Bible says, "as above, so below."

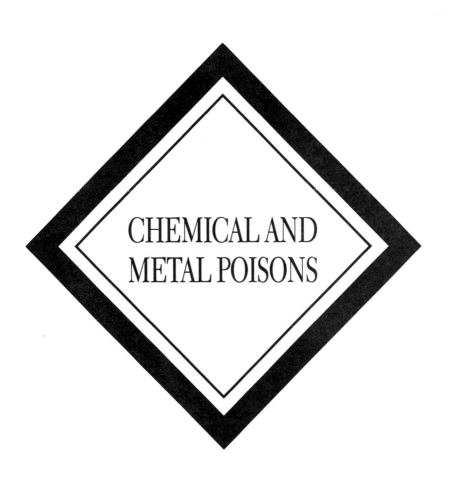

CHEMICAL AND
METAL POISONS

Sodium Fluoride

Our immune systems are constantly under stress. We weaken it further when we brush our teeth with toothpaste containing Sodium Fluoride. Sodium Fluoride is a by-product of the aluminum industry. Because there was an excess of this inexpensive chemical, it was bought up by the pharmaceutical companies and used to replace other more expensive, less harmful forms of fluoride. It is now found in almost all popular toothpaste brands. We do great damage to our bodies when we use this toxic chemical. Each time you brush your teeth, your immune system, your thyroid, parathyroid, thymus and parotid glands are shut down for at least twelve hours. Now if you brush twice daily, you are left totally unprotected. As the sodium fluoride passes through your body it settles and accumulates in the right kidney, where other metal poisons settle, causing kidney problems. Sodium fluoride is also found in the drinking water. While this is not particularly healthy either, this is not nearly as concentrated as it is in toothpaste. There is a way to rebuild after years of using this chemical. First is a tea containing Calendula flowers, Dandelion leaves, Elder flowers, Nettle leaves, Red Root, St. John's Wort and Yarrow flowers. You can buy this tea (called "FRD" or "Fluoride Tea") at any health food store.

Next, after cleaning out the damage, you must rebuild your thyroid and parathyroid glands by using an herbal combination of Yellow Dock, Cleavers, Goldenseal Root, Willow Bark, Club Moss and Uva Ursi. This herb product has a tradename "Metabolizer." For more information on Fluoride check:

Fluoride: The Aging Factor
By Dr. John Yiamouyiannis

Lead

Lead is a toxic metal that is called by medical experts "one of the most common and persistent neurotoxins in the environment." It has been shown to cause damage at even very low levels. It is found in gasoline vapors, car exhaust, paint, hair dyes, tobacco smoke, and on the solder of tin cans. Every person is affected by it but it is the children who are extremely vulnerable. They seem to absorb a much higher percentage of both inhaled and ingested lead. It causes a wide range of disorders including:

> lack of will power
> fatigue
> lack of abstract thinking
> allergies
> anemia
> headaches
> weakness
> hyperactivity in children
> brain dysfunction

Lead causes a wide variety of problems in children and has been marked as one of the leading causes of children with behavioral and learning problems. Lead settles in the brain, nerves, bones and the right kidney. There are three ways to counteract the lead in our system:

1. The herb product "Metaline" which contains pumpkin seed, okra, rhubarb root, capsicum, peppermint and dulse.

2. Homeopathic "Plumbum"

3. This remedy can be made at home and works wonderfully:

    1 gallon cranberry juice

    3 tbsp. whole cloves

    2 tsp. ground cinnamon

    1 tsp. cream of tartar

    Boil the cloves in 1 quart cranberry juice for 20 minutes. Strain and add two tsp. ground cinnamon. Stir and add it to the rest of the cranberry juice. Now add 1 tsp. cream of tartar. Stir. Drink 5 ounces 3 times daily. For children, 3 ounces 3 times daily for 12–15 days. Then do it once a week.

4. Mix these and make a tea and drink 1 cup 3 times daily:

    6 ounces basil

    1 ounce rosemary

    1 ounce hyssop

    1 ounce boneset

5. Red cabbage has been found to help remove lead. Take 1 tablespoon grated red cabbage 3 times daily.

Cadmium

This is another common metal poison. It is also both ingested and inhaled causing a wide variety of symptoms. It is an environmental poison that is found in the water, on our food and in the air. Cadmium is found in processed grains, dairy products, meats, fish, fertilizers, auto exhaust, cigarette smoke, batteries, solder and dentures. It disrupts the absorption of other minerals and tends to settle in the heart and the right kidney. To counteract cadmium poisoning take the

Homeopathic Remedy "Cadmium," increase your zinc intake and use more paprika. According to Naturopathic doctor Stephen R. Schechter, vegetables from the cabbage family also help remove cadmium.

Dioxin

Dioxin is a broad leaf herbicide first widely used in Vietnam. It was one of the ingredients in a product called Agent Orange. It is now commonly used in the United States as a lawn and garden spray and for many commercial uses including the paper manufacturing process. Spraying our lawns causes exposure through both breathing the vapors and playing on the lawn, allowing it to be absorbed through the skin, most commonly through the soles of the feet. We breath it daily in the smog and pollution around industrial cities. It is also commonly found in corn, and is often a factor in people who have corn allergies, causing migraine headaches. Dioxin settles in the brain, the digestive system, and sometimes the kidneys. Dioxin by itself is very toxic, but is usually the cause or the catalyst of many other problems. Dioxin in the body attracts viruses, including Epstein Barr, parasites such as threadworm, whipworm, etc. and many other diseases and syndromes.

God has helped us develop various ways of dealing with this problem. First use the Homeopathic Remedy "Dioxin" to remove it from the body. Next we need to place our food and drink on the "Soma Board" to detoxify it. Finally eat fifteen yellow mustard seeds daily for protection from this poison. It is also helpful to use the "Iron Wire Ring" mentioned in this book to also remove environmental poisons such as dioxin.

Nickel

Nickel is the oxygen robber. It binds with blood fungus and causes tumors. Every tumor needs nickel to hold it together. It has been known to paralyze the spinal column and bring on epilepsy. Nickel is used in industry as a catalyst in the hydrogenation of oils and fats. It is found in margarines as well as oils and fats that are hydrogenated. The Lord provided us with a natural remedy to this poison. Poppy seed removes nickel deposits in two months without side effects. The poppy seed can be taken many ways. It can be taken with rolls, poppy seed cake, and with honey. Take one teaspoon of poppy seeds with honey by mouth twice a day. Also the Homeopathic Remedy "Nickel" is helpful to remove this toxin.

Shower Steam

Tap water contains many dangerous chemicals that form a gas with the shower steam from the hot water. Be careful when breathing steam from tap water with many chemicals added to it. If you feel ill, dizzy, etc., this may be the cause. Use proper ventilation in your bathroom.

Cigarette Smoke

Cigarette smoke is a common source of exposure to radiation and environmental poisons. According to the *New England Journal of Medicine* cigarette smoke contains dangerous levels of:

> lead
> cadmium
> radioactive polonium-210
> radioactive lead
> radium-226
> arsenic

These chemicals have been found in both inhaled and secondary smoke. These chemicals accumulate in the lung and damage delicate tissues. It is estimated that the smoking of 29 cigarettes has an equal exposure to 1 chest X-Ray. In one year, a pack-a-day smoker is exposed to an amount of radiation equal to 300 chest X-Rays. The herb "Calamus Root" has been found to rebuild the lung from smoking damage. Use the following recipe:

> one quart apple juice
> one rounded teaspoon Calamus Root
> Boil both together for 15 minutes, strain, and
> drink six ounces of it, three times daily.

Formaldehyde

Here is a formula Hanna has given to remove formaldehyde from our bodies. Formaldehyde is often present in cheese, milk and sometimes grain.

> 2,000 mg. Vitamin C
> 1 tsp. baking soda
> 100 mg. B-15
> Take this combination 2 times daily for 2 weeks.

Aluminum

Again, unknowingly, we poison ourselves daily. We are attacked from all sides. Aluminum is one of the most common metals found in the earth's crust, always in combination with other elements, forming compounds. It is also an extreme nerve toxin. It builds up in neural tissue, especially the brain, becoming a factor in many diseases including Alzheimer's. Other symptoms of aluminum poison may include: dryness of the mouth, stomach pain, stomach ulcers, hard stool and/or with small hardened pieces ("feces stones"), pain in the spleen area, kidney problems, especially the right kidney, and children will cry a lot. First we must remove the poison from our bodies, and this is done three ways. The first way is by taking the Homeopathic Remedy "Aluminae," second is by taking an herb formula containing pumpkin seeds, okra, rhubarb root, cayenne pepper, red cabbage, and dulse. This product is called "Metaline" and is useful for removing various metals from the body. The third method is by taking a product called "Co Enzyme

International." Also we must remove the metal poisons from the home, and this is often an extensive task. It is more common than you think. First we must remove all the aluminum cooking utensils from the home, including pie tins, pans, wire racks, etc. Now you should avoid drinking from aluminum containers. The aluminum beer can is coated on the inside, but this is not sufficient enough to stop the aluminum from contaminating the beverage. There are many common household items that contain aluminum compounds. The first is antiperspirants. When the Aluminum Chlorohydrate is mixed with alcohol and other chemicals then applied to the sweat glands of the skin, the body all too readily absorbs the aluminum. There are also aluminum compounds found in other products we either ingest or have in our mouth including antacids, baking powder, and toothpaste. Please select these items carefully because brands without aluminum in them do exist and are much safer to use. One last word of caution: The handle on a gasoline pump is made of aluminum and the aluminum even held in the hand nullifies the body's vibration, so when you are filling up the car with gasoline, hold the handle, ideally with a glove, and with the *right* hand, not allowing the aluminum vibration to enter the body. Also don't breathe the vapors from the gasoline; they are full of lead which is harmful.

Mercury

Mercury is a nerve toxin. It settles in the brain, nerves and kidneys. It causes a wide variety of neurological and behavioral disruptions including tremors, uncoordinated movements, deafness, depression, irregular heartbeat, loss of vision, dysphagia and kidney malfunction. Mercury is one of the oldest known common pollutants. Processed mercury has many industrial applications including pesticides, pharmaceutical medicines, cosmetics, dental amalgam fillings, anti-fungal sprays on grains, and batteries. Fifty percent of the mercury used in the U.S. goes into batteries which we commonly dispose of allowing them to decompose in landfills and drain into the soil and ground water. Natural substances used to counteract the effects of mercury include Selenium, which binds with the mercury and allows the body to detoxify itself, and the Homeopathic Remedy "Mercuricum." The herb formula "Metaline" also helps the body counteract the effects of mercury.

Graphite, Nitrates, and Nitrites

These are three lesser known environmental poisons. Nitrates are found in food products like sausage, bacon, meats, hot dogs, and many others. Graphite is an environmental poison found in the air, on our vegetables and food, and around heavy industry. All of these poisons accumulate in the heart causing chest pain and heart malfunction. To remove graphite there is a Homeopathic Remedy "Graphite." To remove nitrate there is an herbal formula called "N.I.T." which works well. It contains Marshmallow Root.

Asbestos

This is a known carcinogen. It usually settles in the lungs. It is found in ceiling insulation and tiles, baby powder, brake shoes of automobiles, and many other commercial uses. Try the Homeopathic Remedy "Asbestos" to remove the damage.

Arsenic

This is a common poison. Many people have arsenic poisoning. It is found in cigarette smoke, pesticides, and dental compounds. Arsenic settles in the muscles. The most common symptom is the constant backache. Having arsenic poisoning causes Chiropractic adjustments not to hold. Other symptoms include constriction of the throat, muscle spasms, low grade fevers, weakness, hair loss, brittle nails, and a garlicky odor to the breath. There is a Homeopathic Remedy called "Arsenicum" which does a terrific job of removing the poison. Again try the herb formula "Metaline." There is also a different way. Raw Mexican Sugar, often called "Piloncillo" in your supermarket. You will find it with the Mexican foods. Take one teaspoon of this sugar three times a day. Break it up into small pieces to make it easier to eat.

ₒld, *Tin, Silver*

..ese are lesser known, not as common environmental toxins. Copper is found in our drinking water due to our pipes.
Tin is found in industrial compounds. Gold and silver are
found in dental structures and in solution in our drinking
water. All have Homeopathic Remedies to relieve any toxic
buildup. For tin, try "Stannum," for gold try "Aurum," for silver try "Argentum," and for copper try "Cuprum."

Drug Watch

The following notice has been paraphrased courtesy of
Gigágeigy's Health Care Management Program:
A tattoo called "Blue Star" is being sold or given to young
school children. It is a small sheet of white paper containing a
blue star, the size of a pencil eraser. Each star is soaked with LSD,
and can be absorbed through the skin by handling the paper.

There are also brightly colored tabs resembling postage
stamps that have pictures of Superman, butterflies, clowns,
Mickey Mouse and other Disney characters on them. These
stamps are packed in a red cardboard box wrapped in foil. This
is a way of distributing LSD or "acid," by appealing to young
children.

A young child could happen upon these and have a fright-
ning or profound emotionally damaging "trip." A child could
iven a tattoo by other children who want to have some fun,
thers who want to cultivate new customers.

A red stamp called "red pyramid" is also being distributed, along with "micro-dot" which comes in various colors. Yet another kind, "window pane" has a grid that can be cut out.

These are all laced with drugs. . . . Please advise your community and your children about these drugs. If you or your child see any of the above, don't handle them. These drugs can react very quickly, and some are laced with strychnine.

Symptoms may include: Hallucinations, nausea, uncontrolled laughter, change in body temperature, mood change (such as fear, or loneliness). If your child has ingested LSD, he or she will be very sensitive to panic, guilt or other emotions. These experiences can leave emotional scars if they are made to be more frightening than necessary. This is not a time to reprimand your child or become upset. Instead be comforting and loving to the child. Contact a poison control center or, if physical symptoms such as vomiting or convulsions occur, take the child to the hospital. Remain calm and present with the child at all times. The effect of the drug could last eight hours or more. The herb Chaparral is useful for removing the damage done by LSD. Take it only for one month at a time then take a break of 3 weeks before starting again.

Iron Wire Ring

There is simple way to remove some of the chemical, metal and environmental poisons, daily, that enter your aura and your body. Use an iron wire, approximately the thickness of a fence wire or a little thicker, to create a circle of about three feet in diameter, leaving one end of the wire pointing out away from the circle, and the other end pointing in toward the center of the circle. Both ends must be directly across the circle, 180° apart. Face both open ends *North* and place the wire ring on the floor. The person in need of cleansing stands facing north also for approximately one minute. As you stand, pray that you are cleared of the poisons and brush down your body. Thank God for this simple and effective remedy.

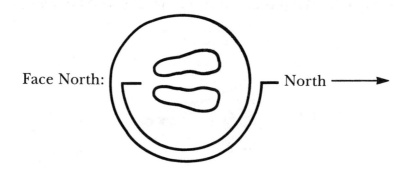

Face North: North ——→

Soma Board

Here is our favorite invention. It's simple to use and effective. The Soma Board was invented to help detoxify poisons left on our food by the use of additives, preservatives, and the grocery scanner. Over a period of time these chemicals can no longer be neutralized by the liver and we are left ill. The vibration created by this small plastic board is enough to neutralize our food and water and make it useful and healthy to the body. It can be taken into restaurants, aboard plane flights, or anywhere you will be eating or drinking. Just place your plate or the food container directly upon the board and allow it to sit for a couple of minutes. Your health will improve tremendously and your energy will return.

Remove Metals Yourself

Here is a way to help yourself. Using your right hand, make a fist and leave your thumb out, pointing up, like a "hitch-hiker." Next, turn your fist toward your chest and press your knuckles into your thymus area in the middle of your sternum. Let your thumb press against your thyroid, located directly on your "Adam's Apple."' Stay in this position for one minute, praying and asking that the metal poisons will be removed.

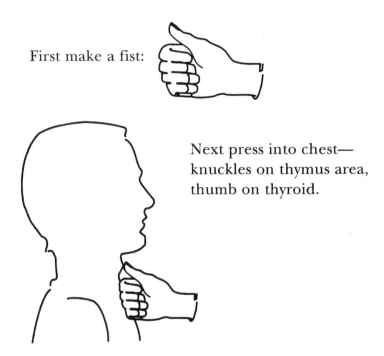

First make a fist:

Next press into chest—
knuckles on thymus area,
thumb on thyroid.

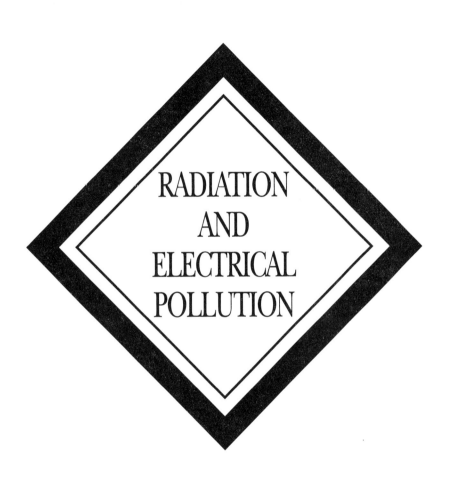

RADIATION
AND
ELECTRICAL
POLLUTION

Fallout

Radioactive chemicals released from the nuclear power and weapons industry combined with other industrial pollution cause a problem known as fallout. Each day, down through the atmosphere, these pollutants flow, causing a wide variety of symptoms including:

anxiety	extreme tiredness
hysteria	pendulous mood swings
insatiable hunger	hot and cold flashes
extreme nervousness	loss of willpower
feeling of unreality	gastric distress
dizziness and vertigo	extreme headache
rheumatic pains	aches in the joints
hearing problems	memory loss
complete exhaustion	sore throat

This damage is widespread. Fallout affects all of us. It lingers in the vegetables, the plants, on the animals, etc. When it rains or snows, we get extra doses of it. Here are a few of the methods used to counteract fallout:

1. 1 tsp. baking soda
    1 tsp. sea salt
    ½ tsp. cream of tartar
    1 quart water
   Mix and drink eight ounces every two hours.

2. Willow leaf tea will help remove the symptoms.

3. Take one piece of bread and toast it dark, burn it. Spread butter over it and sprinkle well with cinna-

mon. Children will enjoy it with a little brown sugar added to it. The combination of the cinnamon and the charcoal (burnt toast) removes fallout.

4. Three Tbsp. baking soda, one Tbsp. Borax. Mix and take ½ teaspoon before meals in 4 ounces water.

5. Homeopathic "R.A. Fallout."

6. According to Dr. Carl C. Pfeifer, to help overcome pollution he recommends this combination of nutrients taken together:
   Lysine
   Cystine
   Methionine

7. After the nuclear accident in Russia vitamin B-15 was given to the population to counteract the fallout and they had good results with it.

8. The herb combination of Willow leaves, Milksugar, Thyme, and Cinnamon. The tradename is "Pol-X." See your Health Food Store.

9. Also three herbs have been very helpful.
   Ginseng
   Valerian Root
   Passa Flora

It is also known that the Vitamins A, B-Complex, and C are helpful to overcome the effects of fallout and radiation.

Stay Free of Environmental Poisons

Peat moss is a great help in removing environmental pollution like electrical fallout, woodpecker waves, obnoxious rays from the earth, radiation in the form of X-Rays, Cobalt, Strontium 60, Plutonium, Uranium, and Fallout.

Take a 5-pound bag of peat moss bought from a garden supply store. Add 1 pound of kelp and place in open containers throughout the house, in front of the television, on top of kitchen cabinets, or where you think it may be needed. Take this same 5 pounds of peat moss to 1 pound of kelp ratio, and mix up enough to place in flat boxes on the floor underneath your bed. A four foot by six foot flat area of peat moss removes the pollution and radiation from the body each night. After six months discard the old mixture, refill the containers with a fresh mixture.

Food Irradiation

There is evidence that genetic, reproductive and other serious health hazards including cancer may be directly linked to the consumption of irradiated foods. Yet, on Feb. 17, 1984, Margaret Heckler, Secretary of the U.S. Dept. of Health and Human Services, announced plans to permit our fruits, vegetables and grains to be exposed to *high* levels of gamma radiation—100,000 to 300,000 rads. That's more than enough to kill living things, including human beings, if they were directly exposed. The idea is to kill insects, bacteria, fungus and viruses, of course. But this is a terribly dangerous idea, a bad idea that will adversely affect the health of everyone in America, unless something is done quickly to prevent this misguided use of nuclear waste products in the food industries.

Since January of 1986, part of the U.S. government plan has been actually in operation: fruits, vegetables and grains can now be subjected to intense gamma rays from Cesium 137 and Cobalt 60. We are already sadly familiar with Cobalt 60 from its use to irradiate people suffering with cancer—we know Cobalt 60's devastating effects on living cells and tissues. What a terrible thing to do to our *food*—merely in the name of extending its "shelf life" in warehouses and at supermarkets.

These radioactive materials come from nuclear power waste products. And the U.S. Dept. of Commerce admits that "food irradiation plants will substantially reduce the disposal costs of nuclear waste." So we see the real motives are financial, not health-related.

Worse yet, we cannot even protect ourselves and our families through reliable labels on the irradiated foods. Only some raw foods are required to be marked "picowaved." But the flour in our bread, for instance, because it is merely an ingredient among others will be completely exempt from proper labeling. There will be no warning that ingredients have been previously exposed to powerful gamma rays. All the dangers of radiolytic products (radiation mutations and toxins) can be in our baked goods, ice cream, T.V. dinners, mixed vegetables and elsewhere—and all with FDA approval!

These are dangers almost unimaginable—of cancerous lesions, kidney disorders, diabetes; of chemical, viral, fungal and other assaults and insults to ourselves and our families. We must act now to overcome the dangers posed by this completely misguided technology and to reverse the unwise Federal policies that are imposing these dangers against all good reason.

Angel Help—Pico Board

This board can be used in conjunction with the Soma Board. They can be placed side by side for a very effective combination. Working as an entire congregation the Chapel of Miracles developed this board to counteract the side effects of food irradiation. Place your food-filled plate on the herb-filled Pico Board. Let it sit for one minute. The food will be free of irradiation.

Remove X-Ray Damage

This is a method to remove the effects after having an X-Ray. Medical X-Rays have exposed more people to dangerous ionizing radiation than both the nuclear power industry and the weapons industry. Oftentimes X-Rays are needed. They have saved countless lives yet the harmful effects of medical X-Rays are greatly underestimated. Always make sure the X-Rays are necessary and as much safety as possible is being used to allow you to be exposed to as little radiation as possible. After the X-Ray use this method to help counteract the damage. Fill a paper sack with equal parts of baking soda and sea salt and rub the bag over the affected area for a couple of minutes. This only has to be done one time. Discard salt and soda afterward.

Salt and Soda Bath

This bath is designed to remove the harmful effects of radiation, fallout, and environmental poisons from the body. Hanna has taught this for years and it is also discussed in the book *Fighting Radiation* by Steven Schechter. Take one pound of sea salt and one pound of baking soda and place into your bath water. Soak for 20 minutes. We have added a new method to this bath. Usually when someone is ill with fallout, radiation poisoning or environmental poisoning, everything in their lives seems out of balance. They become ill, frustrated, nervous, tired and cross.

American Indian Method

We added a technique taught by the American Indians. When the Indian felt upset, nervous, out of balance, he would use this to help himself. He will enter a knee-high, crystal-clear, slow-moving stream, allowing the stream to rush past his feet, knees and ankles. Facing upstream he would bless the water and pray until he comes in contact with the Great Spirit. He would now bend down and with handfuls of water bathe himself, washing each body part. As he did so, he would picture the troubles leaving, being washed away downstream. Each area would be washed, his head would be cleansed of negative thoughts, fear, anguish, his hands cleaned and blessed to do the Great Spirit's work, his back washed clean of pain and troubles. His heart washed and filled with love, hope, strength and joy. As he left, he saw his troubles washed downstream freeing him and allowing him to be back in touch with his world. We can do the same thing. Use your bath water, cleaning and blessing each body part as you wash away illness and disease. Affirm your health and well being knowing that you are truly in touch with God. Drain the tub and watch your troubles leave, never to return.

Clorox Bath

This is an alternative to the salt and soda bath. You now add 6 tablespoons of Clorox to your bath water instead. Be careful. Not everyone can handle Clorox, so check first by letting your feet soak. ← how will you know ?

Radon

According to the U.S. Environmental Protection Agency, long-term exposure to radon gas is the second leading cause of lung cancer, causing as many as 30,000 deaths per year in America. Radon is a radioactive gas given off when uranium decays or breaks down into radium and eventually into radon gas. This gas enters the home through cracks in basement walls and around loose fitting pipes. Once in the lung, the radon, along with a product called radon daughters, emit alpha radiation causing cellular damage. In 1987 the E.P.A. announced that radon may pose a serious threat in eight million U.S. homes. Protecting your home from excess radon gas is done by sealing up cracks and allowing for more ventilation of closed areas. Radon can be tested for in your home. Many companies make effective test kits. If you are suffering from lung difficulties this might be a topic worthy of investigation.

Counteract it by putting 2 teaspoons liquid Chlorophyll in 6 ounces water. Take 500 mg Vitamin C with it. Do this 3 times daily for one week. The same recipe will also remove CARBON MONOXIDE POISON.

Smoke Detectors

This is another source of ionizing radiation in the home. Many of them contain the radioactive products americum, radium, and plutonium. There are brands of smoke detectors on the market that are photoelectric and do not emit such harmful radiation. Always check when buying a specific brand and try to avoid any unnecessary hazards.

Electric Power Lines

Much research is being done on the effects of electric power lines emitting E.L.F., extremely low frequency waves, and damaging our health. Living within 50 feet or so of the lines causes physical and spiritual damage. It is best to avoid moving into an area where the lines are present, but if you are already living or working by these power lines you must protect and heal yourself with a device called the "Computer Pillow." by placing the pillow underneath your feet, on your lap, or behind your back for a few minutes a day, you are able to neutralize the damaging effects these waves have on your body. Computer pillows are herb-filled pillows, which neutralize toxins.

Woodpecker Waves

In addition to the E.L.F. waves that are produced here in our own country, we are continuing to be bombarded with waves from other countries for military purposes. Each day the United States is a target for Soviet Phase Conjugate Weapons that include the "Time Reversed Electromagnetic Wave," the "E.L.F. wave," and the "Woodpecker wave." The waves cause enormous problems by themselves but they can also be used as a vehicle for biological warfare materials. This is a new and important topic and protection is extremely difficult. Undoubtedly new research will be coming in as it is made more available. In order to protect your home from these waves you need two aluminum pie tins. The first one is filled with sea salt and placed on the ceiling in the middle of your home. The second one is hung on the Northwest corner of the house facing toward the center of the house. Personal protection is accomplished by using the methods discussed later in this book.

Microwaves

One of the most damaging devices in your home is the microwave oven. It ruins the vibration of the food cooked in it, making the good unusable and damaging to our bodies. Even more important are the waves it gives off. These concentrated waves extend from the oven filling your home. All family members are affected but the people most injured by this device are the men. The vibration of the waves are most harmful to the male organs and this is so important to the younger boys. A boy raised in a home with a microwave oven has constant problems and will fail to develop properly and to his full potential. The mothers who use these ovens are doing extreme damage to their families. Often times housewives complain about getting rid of their fancy appliance. Do they feed their family out of love, health, happiness, working to build a strong family or do they cook out of obligation and resentment creating a house of ill health and ill feelings. The popularity and convenience should never justify the use of this machine. The choice is simple, the health of yourself and your family or your fancy microwave oven.

Television

The television can also create negative radioactive waves. These waves are easier to control. Crystals can absorb and transmute different types of energies and vibrations. Take Quartz crystals and place them on top and in front of the T.V. The crystals don't have to be large, but they do need to be cleaned periodically. Just take the crystal and set it into a solution of sea salt and water and let it soak overnight. The next day place it back in front of the T.V.

Electric Clock

Sleeping at night with an electric alarm clock close to your bedside also damages your aura. The worst offenders are the clocks with the red L.E.D. numbers on them. Move your alarm clock away from your bedside and you will sleep more comfortably.

Computers

The electromagnetic radiation given off by the computer is also harmful. These waves are most damaging to females. Women working in front of computer terminals need to take extra precautions, especially if they are pregnant. Again, using the "Computer Pillow" will help. Place the pillow on your lap or behind your back, and you will feel more relaxed and comfortable while working on the computer.

Electric Blankets

When we sleep our aura rests. Our circulatory system and our lymphatic system also relaxes. When we use an electric blanket to warm our beds during the night, we do great damage to our aura, and to our blood and lymph transport systems. The vibration of the electricity running through the blanket never allows our aura to rest, and we develop holes in it, which can leave us open to physical and spiritual difficulties. This is the same with our blood and lymph system. All blood diseases, such as leukemia or cancer, are worsened or magnified by using the electric blanket.

Waterbeds

Underneath the waterbed is an electric heater, much like the electric blanket discussed above. The water in the bed is vibrating with the current running through the heater. The heater in the waterbed causes the same problems as the electric blanket. The water in the bed is dangerous also. The water attracts and holds dark forces that attack us when we sleep. The bed itself does not allow the spine to stretch and unravel as it normally would. Although some back problems are relieved as often advertised, there is visually a different and more damaging effect to the very important spinal fluid.

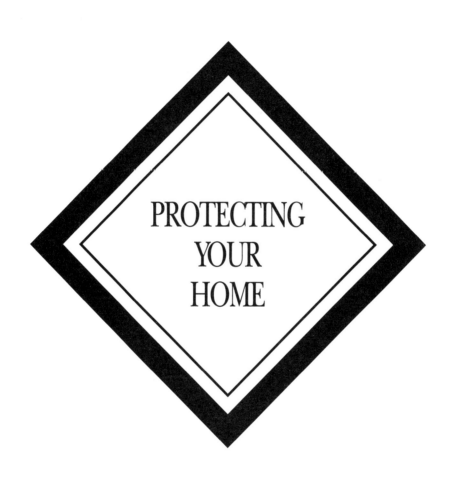

PROTECTING
YOUR
HOME

The Four Hangers

There is a way to balance the energies around a building. This will create positive vibration around your house, further protecting your family. Take four regular steel coat hangers and cut the top hook off as shown in the illustration below. Now place the hangers in each corner of the building in one of these two ways: If you place them outside, bury the hangers flat in the ground, with the two cut ends touching the corners. If you decide to place them inside the house, place them flat under the carpet with the two cut ends facing toward the corners of your room.

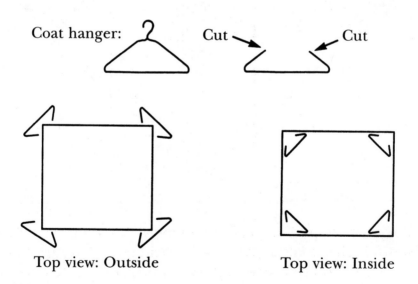

Coat hanger: Cut →   ← Cut

Top view: Outside   Top view: Inside

Balance the Electricity of Your Home

In our homes we have many electrical appliances. The ionic field created by the electricity running through your house and through your appliances needs to be neutralized. In order to do this you can use magnets. Locate the electric meter outside your home. Now just above the meter where the live wires are entering your home, you place this magnetic combination:

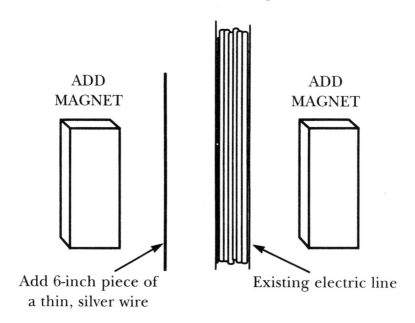

ADD MAGNET   ADD MAGNET

Add 6-inch piece of   Existing electric line
a thin, silver wire

Place two 20 pull magnets, and sandwich a thin, silver wire about 6 inches long against the electric line as in the above illustration. To keep them together, use electrical tape found in your hardware store. The electric current running through your home is now neutralized. What does the magnet do when you put it on the electrical circuit? The wave length of electricity is 23½ inches. The magnet brings the wave length to 3½ inches. This will make the electricity so that it will not do harm to your body.

Full Spectrum Lighting

In order to be healthy and happy we need to spend time each day outdoors, absorbing the sun's rays. The need for sunlight is much the same as our need for food and water. Yet, for many of us, our lifestyles don't allow for the kind of light we need. Now there is a way to recreate the sun's rays and make our work indoors much more enjoyable, without as large a sacrifice of health. "Full Spectrum Lighting" recreates or almost duplicates the wide range of light of the sun. Its intensity level is basically safe and even more consistent in intensity than the sun. Although nothing yet really matches the sun, this is a big improvement over incandescent and fluorescent lighting.

Noise Pollution

Many people live or work in environments with a large amount of noise. This can add to our stress level creating many problems. Noise pollution does cause definite damage to the arterial system. So if you are subjected to continual noise pollution make arrangements to remedy the situation and keep a close eye on your arterial system.

Water

Water is an important part of the cells. It serves as the medium of transport or the carrier for vitamins, minerals, and all of the materials in the blood stream. It serves as a lubricant for your joints and your digestive system. Our bodies are 90% water so it is essential to drink at least 6–8 glasses of pure, clean mineral rich water a day. Obtaining safe healthy drinking water can be a problem. The water that sits in the pipes of your home absorbs metal poisons from the pipes and lead joints. So it is important to run the water a few minutes first thing in the morning in order to get safe water. The water is still filled with some harmful chemicals. The next step is to place the water on the "soma" and "Pico-Angel Help" boards. Many people are now using ozone gas or hydrogen peroxide to purify this water. There is a natural spiritual way to oxygenate and energize our liquids. Simply take the liquid, water, tea, juice, etc. and aerate it by pouring it from container to another container, while blessing the liquid. Now your water has a more positive healthful vibration.

Protect Your Bed

Underneath your house and your bed can be harmful streams of negative energy. This can be a deep-seated under-earth water crossing, electrical wires or Radon gas. They are most harmful to us when we are sleeping. In order to protect ourselves we must place a copper wire around the bed. This is usually easiest attaching it to the box spring. You must start and finish with both ends at the north side of the bed. The starting end of the wire is facing up, toward the ceiling, the finishing end is facing toward the floor. It does not matter which end is up or down, just as long as one is facing up, the other down, both on the north side.

Top view:

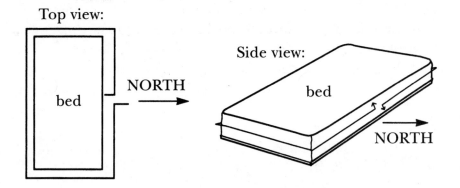

Side view:

Protect Your Trees

Here is a method of protecting your trees given to us by a Minnesota farmer. Take heavy copper wire and on the south side of the tree, drive one end into the ground at least two feet. Next wrap the wire clockwise around the tree 2½ times (you will end up on the north side). Take the end on the north side and allow it to face upward, toward the top of the tree. This will help the tree survive some of the more extreme frosts and protect if from most bugs and pests.

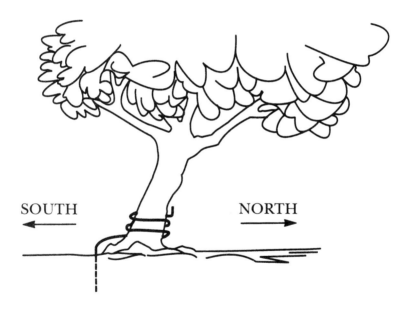

SOUTH ←   NORTH →

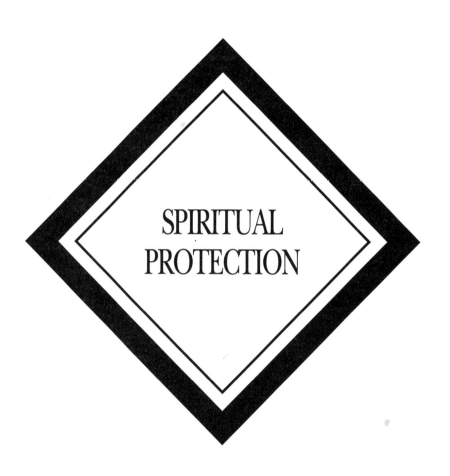

SPIRITUAL
PROTECTION

We live in the age of science. During the past century, unbelievable strides have been made in science and technology. Living in this "high tech" world makes it easy for us to forget our roots, our heritage, our church, and our religion. We awake in the morning feeling rushed and busy, and often times neglecting our spiritual base. Our spiritual bodies and our homes are left unprotected. We have fancy security systems, dead bolt locks, and bars on our windows, yet we leave the spiritual side of our homes and families open to any attack from invaders and dark forces that want to enter. Ignorance and apathy to this situation can cause many problems that can be easily and inexpensively corrected restoring our dark, cold house into a warm, safe, loving home.

The 91st Psalm

The 91st Psalm is for protection. Open your favorite Bible to this Psalm and take some time to recopy it onto a sheet of paper. Write it out; your vibration is in your handwriting and this adds to the protection. Now place the written copy of this Psalm over your door on the inside of your house. People leaving your home have to pass under this, and they leave protected. People entering are protected also. Your home is safeguarded against problems created by dark forces.

Blessing Your City

Our cities are becoming overrun with dark forces. We must stop the hold that gangs, crime and other problems have on our city. Here is how you can spiritually help this problem. You will need seven people. Take the phone book of the area you would like to help and have each person place their right hand palm down over the book. Do not touch each other's hands. Their left hand is out, palm up, open to receive Christ's power. You will all bless the city, asking that every person, building, company, be protected.

Sage

This was the herb used by the American Indians to protect their homes. They also used it to protect themselves in the process called **smudging.** It is usually mixed with other herbs and tied into a bundle or stick, and then burned. The smoke given off is very helpful for cleansing and protecting.

Rock Salt, Alae (Red) Salt and Anise

Dark forces gather in the corners of your home. Round structures are more protected against these dark forces. The Indians knew this and felt safe and content in their round teepees and ceremonial kivas. We can be protected also by using a mixture of special salts and anise. The salts carry the

Christ vibration. When you remove dark forces from your home you should open a door or a window close to the last corner you work on, leaving a place for them to exit. Take the salts into your left hand and bless them with your right hand. Now sprinkle the salts throughout your home. Take a mixture of the salts and the herb anise and place into a small bag. Set these bags into the corners of your home.

In addition to the spiritual protection this mixture provides, it also gives an environmental uplift and releases muscle spasms. The salts act as a crystal, amplifying what they're paired with. The anise acts as a calmative. As a combination it opens and uplifts.

You can buy a pre-made mixture in the form of a pillow in various sizes for your body and also pouches for the corners of rooms. Please refer to the address in the back of this book.

The Mirror

People entering your home often have some entity attached to them. To keep the entity from entering your home, place a small mirror close to the entrance of your house, around or on the door so visitors will look into it when entering. By doing this, the entity will have to stay behind, outside the home, leaving your guests comfortable and happy inside.

Eucalyptus Oil

This oil is great for warding off unwanted entities and dark forces. It's great protection for your home. Whenever you feel the need for some extra help, open a bottle of the oil and place around the home, or around your family. A few drops placed into your bath water is also very effective.

Mistletoe

Mistletoe, like eucalyptus, is also effective against dark forces. It can be placed in a small bag above the door of your home, next to your 91st Psalm to add to the protection, or at various places around your home.

Personal Protection

There are various mixtures that are effective in protecting us personally from the dark forces. They can be placed in small bags and carried on us or placed next to our beds, in our cars, etc. A few of the favorites are:

A. 1 part sea salt
    1 part sand
    1 part cinnamon
    1 part sulphur

B. 4 Tablespoons Epsom Salt
    4 Tablespoons Sea Salt
    2 Tablespoons Sugar
    1 Tablespoon Sulphur
    (You can usually buy Sublimed Sulphur at a drug store.)

C. 4 parts Asa Foetida = (Aspidita)
    3 parts Lobelia
    12 parts Spikenard
    5½ parts Cayenne

None of these are to be taken internally. Just keep them with you or around your home.

Redwood Cross

These next two ideas were given by Klaus Kroeger. Almost all grocery stores use the red laser scanner to price our food. The vibration given off by this scanner is extremely harmful. Inside the Soma Board is material specifically for neutralizing the effects of this scanner. Here is also a different way to keep it from affecting your family once the groceries are into the kitchen. Make a simple six-inch high cross out of the inner bark of a redwood tree and keep it on your kitchen table. The redwood bark is often difficult to obtain but its presence neutralizes these dark forces.

The Feather

Feathers from a peaceful bird carry a very blessing vibration. They are useful when placed under your bedroom pillow, making for a more peaceful sleep. Make sure you use the feather from a peaceful bird, not a hawk or an eagle. Their energies are best used for other purposes.

Praying Over Food

Always remember to give thanks for your food. As you pray over your food, ask that all poisons and toxins be neutralized, and through your prayer the vibration of the food changes and the poisons are released.

9 9 5

There is a combination of numbers that when repeated out loud brings on the vibration of Mother Mary. Use it when you bless food, people, places, etc. Move your right hand in a clockwise circle and with each circle say each number in order:

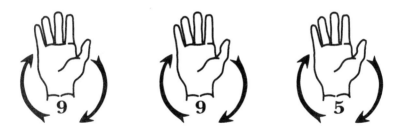

Breaking Bread

When Jesus served or ate bread, he always broke each piece off. By doing so he increased the vibration of this food. We can do the same thing and it works for us also. Whenever you eat a slice of bread, bless is, then break it and the bread will have a positive vibration and will be much healthier.

Help from the Bible

Isaiah 53:5   For healing, say three times in a row, three times daily: "By his stripes thou shall be healed."

Ezekiel 16:6   Repeat three times to stop bleeding.

Psalm 142:5   This Psalm protects us from a dangerous viroid that is rapidly being spread around. A viroid is an infectious particle 150 times smaller than a virus. They can cause extreme illness. Write this Psalm out and carry it with you, the vibration of the written word protects you.

Psalm 58   Use this to break up dark forces.

Psalm 48   This is the antidote for Epstein-Barr.

Mustard Seeds

Yellow mustard seeds serve as protection against Dioxin, Epstein-Barr virus, the AIDS virus, and many others. Each day swallow 15 yellow mustard seeds for males, and 10 for females and you will have some extra protection. Do not overlook this quick and simple technique.

Crystal Laser

This product was developed to enhance the immune system. Every family member should use it each morning for a minute before starting the day. Shine the flashlight over your thymus gland, in the middle of your chest, on your breast bone. This gives your thymus gland and your immune system the extra protection it needs to withstand the daily poisons, wear and tear it can be subjected to. The Crystal Laser gives you a positive attitude toward life, it strengthens the power of positive thinking, it strengthens the immune system, and when the thymus gland and immune system are strengthened, flu, colds, and viral infections will be lessened or eliminated.

Miracle Ring

The energy of the universe, the Christ energy, often times needs to enter our home and become focused at one specific point such as above our desks, our beds, etc. In order to accomplish this, Hanna has a device called the "Miracle Ring." It's an eight-pointed star that hangs from the ceiling. Each point on the star is a triangle, and all eight triangles are different colors, all attached together to form a circle. On top of the ring is a copper strip, a looped coil that is the key part of the Miracle Ring. This whole device is hung from the ceiling over the area where you need the extra energy. Hanna has them hung in her church, above the prayer basket, above her desk and at various places around her Retreat. The rings can be made yourself or ordered through New Age Foods in Boulder.

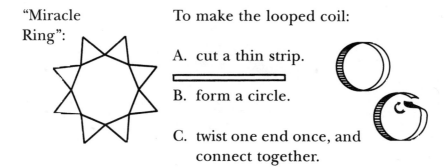

"Miracle Ring":

To make the looped coil:

A. cut a thin strip.

B. form a circle.

C. twist one end once, and connect together.

Hang the coil above the ring, about 2–3 inches, and then hang the whole device in your home.

Shoe Magnets

The dark forces have many, many ways of manipulating our energies. We must work to protect ourselves. Hanna developed a method to eliminate some of the negative energy. Go to your hardware store and buy magnetic tape about ½ inch wide and cut out two one-inch pieces. Place one magnet into the arch of each shoe, sticky side down. You may place it underneath the lining of the shoe if it will make it more comfortable for you.

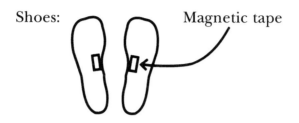

Tags

Hanna has warned us of the tags found in some clothing and on the back of certain brands of wallpaper. On the back side of the tags in some clothes and wallpaper is a pattern of wave lines. She taught us that these lines form a marker or a point of attachment for negative energies or dark forces to keep track of you. Check your clothing and any new wallpaper and if anything looks unusual or unnecessary, either remove the tags or don't buy the product.

Cross Your Arms

There is a method to protect yourself when someone is openly performing exorcisms, removing entities, possessions, etc., and allowing them to freely move onto someone else or gather in the room. Cross your arms covering your chest area. This will hopefully protect you from allowing any of these energies to attach to you.

Here are some addresses concerning literature about environmental toxins:

Making the Switch—Alternatives to Using Toxic Chemicals in the Home
    Publication Dept. $6.00
    Local Government Commission
    909 12th Street, Suite 205
    Sacramento, California 95814

    Sierra Club
    730 Polk Street
    San Francisco, California 94159

    National Coalition to Stop Food Irradiation
    Box 59-0488
    San Francisco, California 94159

    Greenpeace, U.S.A.
    1611 Connecticut Avenue, N.W.
    Washington, D.C. 20009

    Environmental Action
    1525 New Hampshire Avenue, N.W.
    Washington, D.C. 20036

Nontoxic and Natural: The Nontoxic Home
    Debra Lynn Dadd $11.95
    P.O. Box 1506
    Mill Valley, California 94942

Office of Civilian Radioactive Waste Management
Department of Energy
1000 Independence Avenue, S.W.
Washington, D.C. 20585

Nuclear Regulatory Commission
Division of Waste Management
Office of Nuclear Material Safety and Standards
1717 H Street, N.W.
Washington, D.C. 20535

The President
The White House
1600 Pennsylvania Avenue, N.W.
Washington, D.C. 20500
(202) 456-1414

The Vice President
Executive Office Building
Washington, D.C. 20501
(202) 456-2326

You can send telegrams to the White House through any Western Union office for about $5.00.

For the Rock Salt, Alae (Red) Salt and Anise Pillow, contact:

Mary Ellen Turner
3258 South Dale Court
Englewood, Colorado 80110
(303) 789-4078

For spiritual needs and summer retreat classes contact:

Chapel of Miracles
7075 Valmont Drive
Boulder, Colorado 80301
(303) 442-2490

For implements and kits mentioned, including a ready-made mag-net kit to balance the electricity in your home, contact:

Hanna's Herb Shop
5684 Valmont Road
Boulder, Colorado 80301

Books by Hanna

"Wholistic health represents an attitude toward well being which recognizes that we are not just a collection of mechanical parts, but an integrated system which is physical, mental, social and spiritual."

Ageless Remedies from Mother's Kitchen
You will laugh and be amazed at all that you can do in your own pharmacy, the kitchen. These time tested treasures are in an easy to read, cross referenced guide. (92 pages)

Allergy Baking Recipes
Easy and tasty recipes for cookies, cakes, muffins, pancakes, breads and pie crusts. Includes wheat free recipes, egg and milk free recipes (and combinations thereof) and egg and milk substitutes. (34 pages)

Alzheimer's Science and God
This little booklet provides a closer look at this disease and presents Hanna's unique, religious perspectives on Alzheimer's disease. (15 pages)

Arteriosclerosis and Herbal Chelation
A booklet containing information on Arteriosclerosis causes, symptoms and herbal remedies. An introduction to the product *Circu Flow*. (14 pages)

Cancer: Traditional and New Concepts
A fascinating and extremely valuable collection of theories, tests, herbal formulas and special information pertaining to many facets of this dreaded disease. (65 pages)

Cookbook for Electro-Chemical Energies
The opening of this book describes basic principles of healthy eating along with some fascinating facts you may not have heard before. The rest of this book is loaded with delicious, healthy recipes. A great value. (106 pages)

God Helps Those Who Help Themselves
This work is a beautifully comprehensive description of the seven basic physical causes of disease. It is wholistic information as we need it now. A truly valuable volume. (196 pages)

Good Health Through Special Diets
This book shows detailed outlines of different diets for different needs. Dr. Reidlin, M.D. said, "The road to health goes through the kitchen not through the drug store," and that's what this book is all about. (90 pages)

Hanna's Workshop
A workbook that brings together all of the tools for applying Hanna's testing methods. Designed with 60 templates that enable immediate results.

How to Counteract Environmental Poisons
A wonderful collection of notes and information gleaned from many years of Hanna's teachings. This concise and valuable book discusses many toxic materials in our environment and shows you how to protect yourself from them. It also presents Hanna's insights on how to protect yourself, your family and your community from spiritual dangers. (53 pages)

Instant Herbal Locator
This is the herbal book for the do-it-yourself person. This book is an easy cross referenced guide listing complaints and the herbs that do the job. Very helpful to have on hand. (109 pages)

Instant Vitamin-Mineral Locator
A handy, comprehensive guide to the nutritive values of vitamins and minerals. Used to determine bodily deficiencies of these essential elements and combinations thereof, and what to do about these deficiencies. According to your symptoms, locate your vitamin and mineral needs. A very helpful guide. (55 pages)

New Dimensions in Healing Yourself
The consummate collection of Hanna's teachings. An unequated volume that compliments all of her other books as well as her years of teaching. (150 pages)

Old-Time Remedies for Modern Ailments
A collection of natural remedies from Eastern and Western cultures. There are 20 fast cleansing methods and many ways to rebuild your health. A health classic. (105 pages)

Parasites: The Enemy Within
A compilation of years of Hanna's studies with parasites. A rare treasure and one of the efforts to expose the truths that face us every day. (62 pages)

The Pendulum, the Bible and Your Survival
A guide booklet for learning to use a pendulum. Explains various aspects of energies, vibrations and forces. (22 pages)

The Seven Spiritual Causes of Ill Health
This book beautifully reveals how our spiritual and emotional states have a profound effect on our physical well being. It addresses fascinating topics such as karma, gratitude, trauma, laughter as medicine . . . and so much more. A wonderful volume full of timeless treasures. (142 pages)

Spices to the Rescue
This is a great resource for how our culinary spices can enrich our health and offer first aid from our kitchen. Filled with insightful historical references. (64 pages)

COMPUTER PILLOW
SMUDGE (SAGE)
EUCALYPTUS OIL
MISTLETOE